GUIDE TO INTERMITTENT FASTING FOR SENIORS

A Comprehensive Guide To Sustainable Weight Loss and Improved Well-Being through Timed Eating

ANN BRIGHT

TABLE OF CONTENTS

INTRODUCTION

I know you're probably curious about how intermittent fasting can fit into your life and contribute to your overall health and well-being. You might have heard stories from friends or read articles online about the benefits of fasting, but you're looking for a comprehensive guide created specifically for seniors. Well, you've come to the right place!

As we age, our bodies change, and our nutritional needs evolve. It's important to find strategies that support these changes while promoting good health. Intermittent fasting is one such strategy that has gained a lot of attention for its potential health benefits, including weight loss, improved metabolic health, and even enhanced cognitive function. But let's be clear—this isn't about following a fad or jumping on a trend. This book is about understanding the science behind intermittent fasting, exploring its benefits and challenges, and providing practical advice to help you make informed decisions.

I've always believed that health and wellness should be accessible to everyone, regardless of age. That's why this book is written in simple, easy-to-understand language, with of real-life examples and tips to help you on your journey.

Overview of Intermittent Fasting

What is Intermittent Fasting?

Intermittent fasting is more than just a diet—it's an eating pattern that alternates between periods of eating and fasting. Unlike traditional diets that focus on what you eat, intermittent fasting focuses on when you eat. It's a flexible approach that can be adapted to fit your lifestyle and preferences.

Intermittent fasting has been practiced in various forms for centuries. Many cultures and religions incorporate fasting into their rituals, often for spiritual reasons. However, in recent years, scientists and health enthusiasts have taken a closer look at the benefits of fasting, leading to a surge in its popularity as a health and wellness tool.

When I first heard about intermittent fasting, I was skeptical. It sounded counterintuitive—how could not eating for extended periods be good for you? But after some research and hearing positive stories from friends, I decided to give it a try. I started with the 16/8 method, which involves fasting for 16 hours and eating during an 8-hour window. To my surprise, I found it quite manageable. In fact, I began to notice some positive changes in my energy levels and mood within just a few weeks.

One of my favorite things about intermittent fasting is its flexibility. If you have a busy day or social plans, you can adjust your eating window accordingly. It doesn't require strict calorie counting or eliminating your favorite foods. Instead, it encourages mindful eating and a more balanced approach to nutrition.

In the following chapters, we'll explore the different methods of intermittent fasting, discuss how to get started, and provide practical tips and delicious recipes to support you on your journey. Whether you're intending to lose weight, improve your health, or simply try something new, intermittent fasting can be a powerful tool in your wellness arsenal. So let's get started!

Historical Context

Intermittent fasting might seem like a modern trend, but it actually has deep roots in human history. For thousands of years, humans have practiced fasting in various forms, often without even realizing it. Let's take a journey back in time to understand how intermittent fasting has evolved and why it remains relevant today.

Ancient Practices

Fasting has been a natural part of human existence since our hunter-gatherer days. Early humans didn't have access to food 24/7 like we do now. They hunted and foraged for food, which meant there were times of plenty and times of scarcity. This natural cycle of feast and famine helped our bodies adapt to periods without food, making fasting a built-in aspect of our biology.

Religious and spiritual traditions have also embraced fasting for centuries. Many of the world's major religions, including Christianity, Islam, Judaism, Buddhism, and Hinduism, incorporate fasting into their practices. For example:

- **Ramadan:** Muslims fast from dawn to sunset for a month, refraining from eating and drinking during daylight hours.
- **Lent:** Christians observe a 40-day period of fasting and penitence before Easter.
- **Yom Kippur:** Jews fast for 25 hours during this Day of Atonement.

These religious fasts are not just about abstaining from food; they're often seen as a way to purify the body and mind, demonstrate self-discipline, and draw closer to the divine.

Modern Resurgence

In recent years, intermittent fasting has gained popularity in the health and wellness community. This resurgence can be attributed to a growing body of scientific research highlighting its potential benefits. Researchers have begun to explore how fasting affects our bodies at the cellular level and its impact on overall health.

One of the pivotal moments in the modern interest in fasting was the publication of Dr. Michael Mosley's documentary and book, "The Fast Diet," in 2012. Dr. Mosley introduced the 5:2 method, where you eat normally for five days and restrict calories for two non-consecutive days each week. His work brought the concept of intermittent fasting to the mainstream, sparking curiosity and leading to further studies.

Today, intermittent fasting is practiced by millions of people around the world. It's seen not only as a weight loss tool but also as a way to improve overall health, increase longevity, and enhance mental clarity. Let's look into the benefits of intermittent fasting to understand why it's become such a popular approach.

Benefits of Intermittent Fasting

Intermittent fasting offers a range of benefits that can contribute to better health and well-being. These benefits are supported by scientific research and personal anecdotes from people who have incorporated fasting into their lives. Here are some of the key advantages:

1. Weight Loss and Fat Loss

One of the most common reasons people try intermittent fasting is to lose weight.

By restricting the eating window, you naturally reduce the number of calories you consume. This calorie deficit can lead to weight loss over time. Additionally, fasting helps your body switch from burning glucose for energy to burning stored fat, promoting fat loss.

My friend Carol struggled with her weight for years. She tried numerous diets but found them hard to stick to. When she started intermittent fasting, she was surprised at how manageable it was. By following the 16/8 method (fasting for 16 hours and eating during an 8-hour window), she lost 20 pounds over several months and felt more energetic than ever.

2. Improved Metabolic Health

Intermittent fasting can have a positive impact on various metabolic markers. It helps improve insulin sensitivity, which means your body can use insulin more effectively to regulate blood sugar levels.

This is particularly important for reducing the risk of type 2 diabetes.

Scientific Insight: Studies have shown that intermittent fasting can lower blood sugar levels, reduce insulin resistance, and decrease inflammation. These changes contribute to better metabolic health and lower the risk of chronic diseases.

3. Enhanced Brain Function

Fasting doesn't just benefit your body; it can also improve your brain health. Research suggests that intermittent fasting can boost brain function, enhance cognitive performance, and protect against neurodegenerative diseases.

Scientific Insight: Fasting increases the production of brain-derived neurotrophic factor (BDNF), a protein that supports the growth and maintenance of neurons. Higher levels of BDNF are associated with improved memory, learning, and overall brain function.

4. Longevity and Aging

One of the most exciting potential benefits of intermittent fasting is its impact on longevity. Animal studies have shown that calorie restriction and intermittent fasting can extend lifespans. While more research is needed to confirm these effects in humans, the early results are promising.

Scientific Insight: Fasting triggers cellular repair processes, such as autophagy, where the body cleans out damaged cells and regenerates new ones. This process helps reduce the risk of age-related diseases and may contribute to a longer, healthier life.

5. Reduced Inflammation

Chronic inflammation is linked to numerous health conditions, including heart disease, diabetes, and cancer. Intermittent fasting has been shown to reduce markers of inflammation, promoting overall health.

Scientific Insight: By reducing oxidative stress and lowering levels of inflammatory cytokins, fasting helps protect the body against chronic inflammation and its associated diseases.

6. Simplicity and Flexibility

Unlike many diets that require strict meal planning and calorie counting, intermittent fasting is relatively simple. There are no special foods to buy or complex rules to follow. You can choose an eating window that fits your lifestyle and adjust it as needed.

In summary, intermittent fasting offers a flexible and effective approach to improving health and well-being, especially for seniors. By understanding its historical context and the wide range of benefits it provides, you can make an informed decision about whether it's the right choice for you.

Chapter 1:

Understanding Intermittent Fasting

How Intermittent Fasting Works

Intermittent fasting (IF) is not so much about what you eat, but when you eat. The idea is to cycle between periods of eating and fasting. By doing so, you give your body a break from constant digestion, allowing it to focus on other processes like repairing cells and burning fat.

When you eat, your body spends several hours processing and using the food for energy. During this time, your insulin levels are high, and your body stores excess energy as fat. When you fast, your insulin levels drop, signaling your body to start burning stored fat for energy.

This metabolic switch can help you lose weight and improve your overall health.

One of my uncles named Bob was having high sugar levels but was initially skeptical about intermittent fasting when i told him about it. He loved his three square meals a day, with plenty of snacks in between. But when his doctor suggested trying IF to manage his weight and blood sugar levels, he decided to give it a shot. Bob started with a 12-hour fasting window, which was manageable for him. Gradually, he extended his fasting period to 16 hours. Within a few months, Bob noticed he had more energy, lost some weight, and his blood sugar levels improved significantly.

Types of Intermittent Fasting

There are several different ways to practice intermittent fasting. The key is to find a method that fits your lifestyle and is sustainable in the long run. Here are some of the most popular types of intermittent fasting:

16/8 Method: The 16/8 method involves fasting for 16 hours each day and eating during an 8-hour window. For example, if you finish your last meal at 8 p.m., you wouldn't eat again until 12 noon the next day. This method is one of the most popular because it's easy to stick to and can fit into most people's daily routines.

5:2 Diet: The 5:2 diet involves eating normally for five days of the week and restricting calories to about 500-600 on the other two days. These two days should not be consecutive, to avoid feeling overly deprived. For example, you might choose to eat a small breakfast and dinner on Monday and Thursday, then eat normally on the other days.

Eat-Stop-Eat: The Eat-Stop-Eat method involves fasting for a full 24 hours once or twice a week. For example, if you finish dinner at 7 p.m. on Monday, you wouldn't eat again until 7 p.m. on Tuesday. During the fasting period, you can drink water, tea, or coffee, but no solid food.

Alternate-Day Fasting: Alternate-Day Fasting (ADF) involves alternating between days of normal eating and days of fasting. On fasting days, you might consume very few calories (about 500) or none at all. This method can be quite effective for weight loss but can also be challenging to maintain long-term.

Intermittent fasting offers a flexible and effective approach to improving health and well-being, especially for seniors. By understanding how intermittent fasting works and exploring different methods, you can find a routine that fits your lifestyle and goals. Remember, it's important to choose a method that you can stick to and that makes you feel good.

The Science Behind Fasting

Intermittent fasting isn't just a trend, it's backed by a significant amount of scientific research that explains why and how it works. Understanding the science behind fasting can help you appreciate its benefits and make informed decisions about incorporating it into your lifestyle. Here, we will look into the key scientific mechanisms that make intermittent fasting effective:

Metabolic Changes:
When you fast, your body undergoes several metabolic changes that can have a profound impact on your health. Here's how it works:

1. **Switching Energy Sources:** Normally, your body uses glucose (sugar) from the food you eat as its primary source of energy. However, when you fast, your body depletes its glucose stores and starts to burn fat for energy. This process is called ketosis. By shifting to fat as a primary energy source, your body becomes more efficient at burning stored fat, which can lead to weight loss.

2. **Increased Growth Hormone Production:** Fasting can increase the levels of human growth hormone (HGH) in your body. HGH plays a crucial role in fat metabolism, muscle growth, and overall health. Higher levels of HGH can help you maintain muscle mass while losing fat, which is particularly important for seniors.

3. **Enhanced Fat Burning:** When insulin levels are low (as they are during fasting), your body can more easily access stored fat and convert it into energy. This is why intermittent fasting can be an effective strategy for reducing body fat.

Cellular Repair Processes:

Fasting triggers various cellular repair processes that can enhance your health and longevity. One of the most important processes is called autophagy.

1. **Autophagy:** During fasting, your cells initiate autophagy, a process where they remove damaged components and recycle them for energy. This helps to clean out cellular debris and improve the function of your cells. Think of it as a cellular housekeeping process

that rejuvenates your body from the inside out.

2. **Reduced Inflammation:** Fasting has been shown to reduce levels of inflammation in the body. Chronic inflammation is linked to many diseases, including heart disease, diabetes, and cancer. By promoting autophagy and reducing inflammation, fasting can help protect against these conditions.

3. **Longevity and Disease Prevention**: Animal studies have shown that fasting can extend lifespan by improving cellular health and reducing the incidence of age-related diseases. While more research is needed in humans, the findings so far are promising.

Insulin Sensitivity:

One of the most well-documented benefits of intermittent fasting is its ability to improve insulin sensitivity, which is crucial for maintaining healthy blood sugar levels.

Insulin's Role: Insulin is a hormone that helps regulate blood sugar levels by facilitating the uptake of glucose into cells. When you eat, your blood sugar levels rise, and your pancreas releases insulin to help transport glucose into your cells for energy.

Insulin Sensitivity vs. Insulin Resistance:

Insulin sensitivity refers to how effectively your cells respond to insulin. High insulin sensitivity means your cells use insulin efficiently, keeping blood sugar levels stable. On the other hand, insulin resistance occurs when your cells become less responsive to insulin, leading to higher blood sugar levels and an increased risk of type 2 diabetes.

How Fasting Helps: Intermittent fasting can improve insulin sensitivity by lowering blood insulin levels and reducing insulin resistance. During fasting periods, your body has a chance to reset its insulin response, making your cells more sensitive to insulin when you do eat. This helps maintain stable blood sugar levels and reduces the risk of metabolic diseases.

Scientific Insight: Studies have shown that intermittent fasting can lead to significant improvements in insulin sensitivity and blood sugar control. For example, a study published in the journal "Cell Metabolism" found that intermittent fasting reduced insulin levels and improved insulin sensitivity in both overweight and obese individuals.

Understanding the science behind intermittent fasting helps to demystify why it works and why it can be such a powerful tool for health and well-being. By promoting metabolic changes, enhancing cellular repair processes, and improving insulin sensitivity, intermittent fasting offers numerous benefits that can contribute to better health, especially for seniors.

Chapter 2:

Benefits of Intermittent Fasting for Seniors

Intermittent fasting (IF) can be particularly beneficial for seniors, offering a range of health benefits that contribute to overall well-being. This chapter will explore how IF can help with weight loss, improve metabolic health, enhance brain function, promote longevity, reduce inflammation, and manage chronic conditions like diabetes, heart disease, and arthritis.

1. Weight Loss

Weight loss is often a primary reason people try intermittent fasting. For seniors, maintaining a healthy weight is crucial for preventing various health issues.

How IF Helps: Intermittent fasting can help reduce overall calorie intake by limiting the eating window. Additionally, fasting periods can boost your metabolism and promote fat burning. The 16/8 method, where you fast for 16 hours and eat during an 8-hour window, is particularly effective for weight loss.

2. Improved Metabolic Health

Metabolic health is vital for seniors, as it influences your energy levels, weight management, and risk of chronic diseases.

How IF Helps: Intermittent fasting improves insulin sensitivity, making your body more efficient at regulating blood sugar levels. It can also lower cholesterol and triglyceride levels, reducing the risk of metabolic syndrome.

Scientific Insight: Studies show that intermittent fasting can lead to significant improvements in metabolic markers. For instance, fasting can lower blood insulin levels, reduce insulin resistance, and promote better blood sugar control.

3. Enhanced Brain Function

As we age, maintaining cognitive function becomes increasingly important. Intermittent fasting can benefit brain health in several ways.

How IF Helps: Fasting can increase the production of brain-derived neurotrophic factor (BDNF), a protein that supports the growth and maintenance of neurons. Higher BDNF levels are associated with improved memory, learning, and overall brain function.

Scientific Insight: Research indicates that intermittent fasting can enhance cognitive performance and protect against neurodegenerative diseases like Alzheimer's and Parkinson's. Fasting promotes the production of ketones, an alternative energy source for the brain that can improve mental clarity.

4. Longevity and Aging

One of the most exciting benefits of intermittent fasting is its potential to promote longevity and healthy aging.

How IF Helps: Fasting triggers autophagy, a process where your body cleans out damaged cells and regenerates new ones. This cellular repair mechanism can help slow down aging and reduce the risk of age-related diseases.

Scientific Insight: Animal studies have shown that intermittent fasting can extend lifespan by improving cellular health and reducing the incidence of age-related diseases. While more research is needed in humans, the initial findings are promising.

5. Reduced Inflammation

Chronic inflammation is linked to many health issues, including heart disease, diabetes, and arthritis. Intermittent fasting can help reduce inflammation and promote overall health.

How IF Helps: Fasting reduces oxidative stress and lowers levels of inflammatory cytokines. This helps protect the body against chronic inflammation and its associated diseases.

Scientific Insight: Studies have shown that intermittent fasting can decrease markers of inflammation. By promoting cellular repair and reducing oxidative stress, fasting helps mitigate the effects of chronic inflammation.

6. Managing Chronic Conditions

Intermittent fasting can be an effective tool for managing various chronic conditions, which are common in seniors. Here's how it can help with diabetes, heart disease, and arthritis:

Diabetes

How IF Helps: Intermittent fasting improves insulin sensitivity and helps regulate blood sugar levels. It can also reduce insulin resistance, a key factor in managing type 2 diabetes.

Scientific Insight: Research has shown that intermittent fasting can lead to significant reductions in blood sugar levels and improvements in insulin sensitivity, making it a powerful strategy for managing diabetes.

Heart Disease

How IF Helps: Intermittent fasting can lower blood pressure, reduce cholesterol levels, and decrease inflammation, all of which are important for heart health.

Scientific Insight: Studies indicate that fasting can improve cardiovascular health by reducing risk factors such as high cholesterol, hypertension, and inflammation.

Arthritis

How IF Helps: Fasting can reduce inflammation, which is a major contributor to arthritis pain and stiffness. By lowering inflammation, intermittent fasting can help alleviate symptoms and improve joint health.

Scientific Insight: Research suggests that intermittent fasting can reduce inflammatory markers, potentially easing symptoms of arthritis and other inflammatory conditions.

Chapter 3:

Getting Started with Intermittent Fasting

Embarking on an intermittent fasting (IF) journey can be exciting and transformative, but it's essential to start on the right foot. This chapter will guide you through determining if IF is suitable for you and how to choose the best fasting method for your lifestyle and goals.

Is Intermittent Fasting Right for You?

Before diving into intermittent fasting, it's important to evaluate whether this approach fits your unique health needs and circumstances.

Consult Your Doctor

Before making any significant changes to your diet or lifestyle, it's crucial to consult your healthcare provider. This is especially true for seniors, as fasting can impact various aspects of health, such as blood sugar levels, medication effectiveness, and overall well-being.

What to Discuss: When talking to your doctor, mention your interest in intermittent fasting and discuss your current health status. Be open about any medical conditions, medications you're taking, and any concerns you might have. Your doctor can provide personalized advice and ensure that fasting won't interfere with your health.

Assess Your Health Status

Evaluate Your Current Health: Take stock of your current health status, including any chronic conditions, medications, and dietary habits. Intermittent fasting can be beneficial for many, but it's not for everyone. Understanding your health baseline will help you make informed decisions and set realistic goals.

Consider Your Lifestyle: Think about your daily routine, social commitments, and personal preferences. Different fasting methods can fit various lifestyles, so choosing one that aligns with your habits and schedule is important.

Choosing the Right Fasting Method

Once you've determined that intermittent fasting is a good fit for you, the next step is to choose the right fasting method. Here are some popular options and tips for selecting the one that suits you best.

16/8 Method

How It Works: The 16/8 method involves fasting for 16 hours each day and eating during an 8-hour window. For example, you might eat from noon to 8 p.m. and fast from 8 p.m. to noon the next day.

Who It's For: This method is great for beginners because it fits easily into most lifestyles. It's also flexible enough to accommodate social events and daily routines.

5:2 Diet

How It Works: The 5:2 diet involves eating normally for five days a week and restricting calorie intake to about 500-600 calories on two non-consecutive days.

Who It's For: This method is suitable for those who prefer more flexibility in their daily eating habits but are okay with two days of low-calorie intake.

Eat-Stop-Eat

How It Works: The Eat-Stop-Eat method involves fasting for a full 24 hours once or twice a week. For example, if you finish dinner at 7 p.m. on Monday, you wouldn't eat again until 7 p.m. on Tuesday.

Who It's For: This method is ideal for those who can handle a full day without food and prefer fewer fasting days.

Alternate-Day Fasting

How It Works: Alternate-Day Fasting (ADF) involves alternating between days of normal eating and days of fasting, where you might consume very few calories (about 500) or none at all.

Who It's For: This method can be quite effective for weight loss but can also be challenging to maintain long-term.

Setting Realistic Goals

Setting realistic and achievable goals is crucial when starting intermittent fasting. Goals give you direction and motivation, helping you stay committed to your new eating pattern.

Understand Your Why: Clearly define why you want to start intermittent fasting. Whether it's for weight loss, improving metabolic health, enhancing brain function, or managing a chronic condition, having a clear purpose will keep you motivated.

Set Specific Goals: Instead of vague goals like "lose weight," set specific ones such as "lose 10 pounds in three months" or "reduce fasting blood sugar levels by 10% in six months." Specific goals are measurable and easier to track.

Be Realistic: Aim for achievable milestones that consider your age, health status, and lifestyle. For instance, a realistic goal might be to gradually extend your fasting period by an hour each week until you reach your desired fasting window.

Track Your Progress: Keep a journal to monitor your progress, noting any changes in weight, energy levels, mood, and health markers. This will help you stay on track and make necessary adjustments.

Be Flexible: Life can be unpredictable, so allow some flexibility in your goals. If you face setbacks, don't get discouraged. Adjust your goals if needed and keep moving forward.

Preparing for the Transition

Transitioning to intermittent fasting can be a significant change, but with proper preparation, you can make the process smoother and more manageable.

Gradual Implementation

Start Slowly: Instead of jumping into a strict fasting schedule, ease into it. Begin with a shorter fasting window, such as 12 hours, and gradually increase it by an hour every few days or weeks until you reach your target fasting period.

Choose the Right Time: Pick a time to start when you don't have major social commitments or stressful events. This way, you can focus on adapting to the new eating pattern without additional pressure.

Adjust Meal Timing: Gradually shift your meal times to align with your chosen fasting window. For example, if you're aiming for a 16/8 schedule, slowly push back your breakfast time while bringing dinner earlier.

Managing Hunger

Stay Busy: Keeping yourself occupied can help distract you from hunger. Engage in activities you enjoy, such as reading, walking, or hobbies, especially during your fasting hours.

Drink Plenty of Water: Hydration is key to managing hunger. Drinking water can help you feel full and prevent dehydration. Herbal teas and black coffee (without sugar or cream) are also good options.

Plan Your Meals: Plan nutritious and satisfying meals for your eating window. Focus on foods high in fiber, protein, and healthy fats, which can help you feel fuller for longer.

Listen to Your Body: Pay attention to your body's signals. If you feel dizzy, extremely hungry, or unwell, it's okay to adjust your fasting schedule or break your fast. Your well-being is the priority.

Gradual Reduction: If you find it difficult to stick to the fasting period, gradually reduce the length of your fasting window and slowly build it back up as your body adjusts.

Staying Hydrated

Importance of Hydration: Staying hydrated is crucial during fasting. Water helps regulate body temperature, maintain energy levels, and support overall health. Dehydration can lead to headaches, fatigue, and difficulty concentrating.

How Much to Drink: Aim for at least 8-10 glasses of water per day. This may vary based on individual needs, activity levels, and climate. Listen to your body and drink when you feel thirsty.

Hydration Tips:
- **Carry a Water Bottle:** Keep a water bottle with you throughout the day to remind yourself to drink.
- **Set Reminders:** Use a phone app or alarms to remind you to drink water regularly.

- **Flavor Your Water:** If plain water is unappealing, add a slice of lemon, cucumber, or a few mint leaves to enhance the taste.

- **Hydrating Foods:** Include hydrating foods like fruits and vegetables in your meals, such as cucumbers, oranges, and watermelon.

- **Avoid Dehydrating Beverages**: Limit intake of caffeinated and sugary drinks, as they can lead to dehydration. Stick to water, herbal teas, and black coffee in moderation.

Chapter 4:

Nutrition and Intermittent Fasting

Proper nutrition is essential when practicing intermittent fasting, especially for seniors. Ensuring you get the right nutrients during your eating windows can enhance the benefits of fasting and support overall health. This chapter covers the essential nutrients seniors need, foods to include and avoid, and the role of supplements and multivitamins.

Essential Nutrients for Seniors

As we age, our nutritional needs change. It's crucial to focus on specific nutrients that support aging bodies and promote optimal health.

Protein

Importance: Protein is vital for maintaining muscle mass, strength, and overall body function. It also helps in repairing tissues, producing enzymes and hormones, and supporting immune function.

Sources: Include lean meats, poultry, fish, eggs, dairy products, beans, legumes, and plant-based proteins like tofu and quinoa. Aim for a balanced intake throughout your eating window to ensure your body gets a steady supply of protein.

Vitamins and Minerals

Importance: Seniors need adequate vitamins and minerals to support various bodily functions and prevent deficiencies. Key vitamins and minerals include:

- **Calcium and Vitamin D:** Essential for bone health. Dairy products, fortified plant milks, leafy greens, and sunlight exposure are good sources.

- **Vitamin B12:** Important for nerve function and red blood cell production. Found in animal products like meat, dairy, and eggs.
- **Magnesium**: Supports muscle and nerve function, blood sugar control, and bone health. Found in nuts, seeds, whole grains, and leafy greens.
- **Potassium:** Helps regulate blood pressure and fluid balance. Found in fruits (bananas, oranges), vegetables (potatoes, spinach), and legumes.
- **Omega-3 Fatty Acids:** Promote heart health and reduce inflammation. Found in fatty fish (salmon, mackerel), flaxseeds, and walnuts.

Foods to Include

Choosing nutrient-dense foods during your eating windows is crucial for getting the most out of intermittent fasting.

1. Whole Foods

Importance: Whole foods are minimally processed and rich in essential nutrients. They provide a balance of vitamins, minerals, and fiber that support overall health.

Examples: Fresh fruits and vegetables, whole grains, nuts, seeds, and legumes. These foods help you feel full longer and provide sustained energy.

2. Healthy Fats

Importance: Healthy fats support brain health, hormone production, and nutrient absorption. They also provide a slow, steady source of energy.

Sources: Avocados, nuts, seeds, olive oil, and fatty fish like salmon and mackerel. Incorporate these fats into your meals to keep you satisfied and support heart health.

3. Lean Proteins

Importance: Lean proteins are essential for muscle maintenance and repair, especially important for seniors to prevent muscle loss.

Sources: Skinless poultry, lean cuts of beef and pork, fish, eggs, dairy products, beans, lentils, and tofu. Ensure you include a source of lean protein in each meal to meet your daily requirements.

4. Complex Carbohydrates

Importance: Complex carbohydrates provide sustained energy and are rich in fiber, which supports digestive health.

Sources: Whole grains (brown rice, quinoa, oats), vegetables (sweet potatoes, carrots), and legumes (beans, lentils). These foods help maintain stable blood sugar levels and keep you full longer.

Foods to Avoid

Certain foods can undermine the benefits of intermittent fasting and negatively impact health, particularly for seniors.

1. Processed Foods

Processed foods are often high in unhealthy fats, sugars, and sodium, and low in essential nutrients. They can contribute to weight gain, inflammation, and chronic diseases.

Examples: Packaged snacks, ready-to-eat meals, fast food, and processed meats (sausages, hot dogs). Opt for whole, unprocessed foods instead.

2. Sugary Snacks

Sugary snacks can cause blood sugar spikes and crashes, leading to energy fluctuations and increased hunger.

Examples: Candy, cookies, cakes, and sugary drinks. Choose natural sources of sweetness like fruits or small amounts of dark chocolate if you crave something sweet.

3. Excessive Refined Carbs

Refined carbohydrates, such as white bread and pastries, lack fiber and essential nutrients. They can cause rapid blood sugar spikes, contributing to weight gain and metabolic issues.

Examples: White bread, pasta, pastries, and sugary cereals. Opt for whole grain alternatives that provide more fiber and nutrients.

Supplements and Multivitamins

While a balanced diet should provide most of the nutrients you need, supplements and multivitamins can help fill any gaps, especially for seniors.

Multivitamins: A daily multivitamin can ensure you're getting essential vitamins and minerals, especially if your diet varies. Look for formulations specifically designed for seniors, which often include higher doses of vitamins D and B12, and calcium.

Calcium and Vitamin D: If you're not getting enough from food and sunlight, consider supplements to support bone health.

Omega-3 Supplements: If you don't consume enough fatty fish, omega-3 supplements can help reduce inflammation and support heart health.

Magnesium: A magnesium supplement can help with muscle function and sleep, particularly if your diet is low in magnesium-rich foods.

Consult Your Doctor: Before starting any supplements, consult your healthcare provider to determine the right dosage and ensure they won't interact with any medications you're taking.

Chapter 5:

Intermittent Fasting for Weight Loss

Intermittent fasting (IF) has gained popularity as an effective strategy for weight loss. This chapter looks into how intermittent fasting aids weight loss and how to create a calorie deficit to maximize results.

How Intermittent Fasting Aids Weight Loss

Intermittent fasting influences weight loss through various mechanisms that impact metabolism, hormones, and calorie intake.

Calorie Restriction: By limiting the time window for eating, intermittent fasting naturally reduces calorie intake.

Fasting periods create a calorie deficit, which is essential for weight loss.

Boosts Metabolism: Contrary to common belief, intermittent fasting can actually boost metabolism. During fasting periods, the body switches to burning stored fat for energy, leading to increased fat oxidation and metabolic rate.

Reduces Insulin Levels: Intermittent fasting improves insulin sensitivity, leading to lower insulin levels. Reduced insulin levels promote fat burning and make it easier for the body to access stored fat for energy.

Increases Growth Hormone Levels: Fasting triggers the release of growth hormone, which plays a key role in fat metabolism and muscle growth. Higher growth hormone levels promote fat loss and preserve lean muscle mass.

Promotes Fat Loss While Preserving Muscle: Unlike traditional calorie restriction diets, intermittent fasting has been shown to promote fat loss while preserving lean muscle mass. This is important for maintaining metabolic health and preventing muscle loss during weight loss.

Creating a Calorie Deficit

Creating a calorie deficit is essential for weight loss, regardless of the dietary approach. Here's how to create a calorie deficit while practicing intermittent fasting:

Calculate Your Basal Metabolic Rate (BMR): Your BMR is the number of calories your body needs to maintain basic physiological functions at rest. There are online calculators available to estimate your BMR based on factors like age, gender, weight, and height.

Determine Your Total Daily Energy Expenditure (TDEE): Your TDEE is the total number of calories you burn in a day, including physical activity. Multiply your BMR by an activity factor (typically 1.2 to 1.9) to estimate your TDEE.

Set a Realistic Calorie Goal: To create a calorie deficit, aim to consume fewer calories than your TDEE. A moderate deficit of 500 to 750 calories per day is generally recommended for sustainable weight loss.

Track Your Caloric Intake: Use a food diary or a calorie tracking app to monitor your daily food intake. Be mindful of portion sizes and the calorie content of foods.

Plan Balanced Meals: Focus on nutrient-dense, whole foods that provide essential nutrients while keeping calories in check. Include plenty of fruits, vegetables, lean proteins, healthy fats, and whole grains in your meals.

Practice Portion Control: Be aware of portion sizes and avoid overeating, even during your eating windows. Pay attention to hunger and fullness cues to prevent excessive calorie intake.

Stay Consistent: Consistency is key to achieving and maintaining a calorie deficit. Stick to your fasting schedule and be mindful of your food choices to stay on track with your weight loss goals.

Be Patient: Weight loss takes time, and progress may not always be linear. Celebrate small victories along the way and stay focused on your long-term goals.

Monitor Progress: Regularly track your weight, measurements, and body composition to monitor your progress.

Adjust your calorie intake or fasting schedule as needed to continue seeing results.

Tracking Your Progress

Tracking your progress is essential for staying motivated and making informed decisions on your intermittent fasting journey. Here's how to effectively track your progress:

1. Set Clear Goals: Define specific, measurable goals related to weight loss, health improvements, or fitness milestones. Having clear objectives will give you something to strive for and help you track your progress more effectively.

2. Use Multiple Metrics: Don't rely solely on the scale to measure progress. Track other metrics like body measurements (waist circumference, hip circumference), body fat percentage, and changes in clothing size. These metrics provide a more comprehensive view of your progress than just weight.

3. Keep a Food Diary: Record your food intake, including portion sizes and meal times, to track your calorie intake and eating patterns. This can help you identify areas for improvement and ensure you're staying on track with your dietary goals.

4. Monitor Physical Activity: Keep track of your exercise routine, including the type of activity, duration, and intensity. Regular physical activity complements intermittent fasting for weight loss and overall health, so monitoring your workouts can help you stay accountable and track improvements in fitness levels.

5. Take Progress Photos: Periodically take photos of yourself from different angles to visually track changes in your body composition over time.

Sometimes changes in body composition may not be reflected on the scale, but progress photos can provide visual evidence of your transformation.

6. Track Non-Scale Victories: Celebrate small victories and improvements in energy levels, mood, sleep quality, and overall well-being. These non-scale victories are just as important as changes in weight and can keep you motivated during your journey.

Overcoming Weight Loss Plateaus

Weight loss plateaus occur when your weight remains steady despite continuing efforts to lose weight through diet and exercise. This can be a frustrating and demotivating experience, but it's a common part of the weight loss journey including intermittent fasting.

Causes of Weight Loss Plateaus

1. **Metabolic Adaptation**: As you lose weight, your body's metabolism slows down to conserve energy. This is a natural survival mechanism that can make further weight loss more challenging.

2. **Loss of Muscle Mass**: During weight loss, you may lose muscle as well as fat. Since muscle burns more calories at rest than fat, losing muscle can decrease your overall calorie expenditure.

3. **Caloric Intake Adjustments**: As your body weight decreases, your caloric needs also decrease. Continuing to consume the same number of calories can lead to a plateau.

4. **Body's Set Point**: Your body has a natural weight range, known as a set point, where it feels comfortable. When you approach

this range, weight loss may slow down or stop.

5. **Inconsistent Eating Habits**: Occasional overeating or underestimating calorie intake can prevent further weight loss.

6. **Lack of Variety in Exercise**: Doing the same workouts repeatedly can lead to a plateau as your body becomes efficient at performing those exercises, burning fewer calories.

Here's how to overcome them:

1. Reassess Your Caloric Intake: As you lose weight, your calorie needs may decrease, so it's essential to adjust your calorie intake accordingly. Recalculate your TDEE and adjust your calorie deficit if necessary to continue making progress.

2. Mix Up Your Fasting Routine: Experiment with different fasting schedules, meal timing, or fasting methods to keep your body guessing and prevent adaptation. Consider incorporating occasional longer fasts or alternate-day fasting to shake things up.

3. Focus on Nutrient Density: Ensure your meals are nutrient-dense and provide essential vitamins, minerals, and macronutrients. Focus on whole, unprocessed foods that fuel your body and support overall health.

4. Increase Physical Activity: Ramp up your exercise routine to boost calorie expenditure and stimulate fat loss. Incorporate a combination of cardiovascular exercise, strength training, and flexibility exercises for optimal results.

5. Manage Stress: High stress levels can hinder weight loss progress by increasing cortisol levels, which can promote fat storage, particularly around the abdomen. Practice stress-reducing techniques like meditation, deep breathing, yoga, or spending time in nature.

6. Be Patient and Persistent: Weight loss plateaus are normal and temporary. Stay committed to your plan, trust the process, and be patient with yourself. Focus on making sustainable lifestyle changes rather than chasing rapid weight loss.

Maintaining Weight Loss

Maintaining weight loss can be challenging, but with the right strategies, it's possible to sustain your progress long-term:

1. Establish Healthy Habits: Focus on building healthy habits that support weight maintenance, such as regular exercise, balanced nutrition, adequate sleep, stress management, and mindful eating.

2. Practice Moderation: Enjoy your favorite foods in moderation and be mindful of portion sizes. Avoid extreme or restrictive diets that are difficult to maintain over the long term.

3. Stay Active: Continue to prioritize regular physical activity to support weight maintenance, muscle retention, and overall health. Find activities you enjoy and make them a regular part of your routine.

4. Monitor Your Progress: Keep track of your weight and other key metrics regularly to catch any changes early and make adjustments as needed. Regular monitoring can help you stay accountable and prevent significant weight regain.

5. Stay Consistent: Consistency is key to maintaining weight loss. Stick to your healthy habits, even when life gets busy or challenging. Remember that small, consistent efforts over time lead to significant results.

6. Seek Support: Surround yourself with a supportive network of friends, family, or online communities who understand your goals and can provide encouragement, accountability, and motivation.

7. Celebrate Your Successes: Celebrate your achievements and milestones along the way. Recognize and reward yourself for your hard work and dedication to maintaining a healthy lifestyle.

Chapter 6:

Intermittent Fasting and Overall Well-Being

Intermittent fasting not only impacts physical health but also plays a significant role in promoting overall well-being. It offers a range of mental health benefits, including reduced stress and improved mood. By regulating stress hormones, enhancing stress resilience, and promoting neurochemical balance in the brain, intermittent fasting can positively impact mental well-being. Incorporating intermittent fasting into your lifestyle can contribute to a healthier mind-body connection and enhance your overall quality of life.

Mental Health Benefits

Intermittent fasting has been associated with various mental health benefits that can contribute to overall well-being and quality of life.

1. Reduced Stress

Stress Reduction: Intermittent fasting can help reduce stress levels by lowering cortisol, the body's primary stress hormone. During fasting periods, cortisol levels tend to decrease, leading to a calmer physiological state.

Enhanced Stress Response: Fasting may improve the body's response to stress by increasing resilience and adaptability. Research suggests that intermittent fasting can activate cellular stress response pathways, which may confer protective effects against chronic stress.

Improved Stress Management: Practicing intermittent fasting can promote mindfulness and self-awareness around eating habits, which can translate to better stress management skills. Learning to navigate hunger cues and food cravings during fasting periods can empower individuals to cope with stress more effectively.

2. Improved Mood

Regulation of Neurotransmitters: Intermittent fasting may influence neurotransmitter activity in the brain, including serotonin and dopamine, which play key roles in regulating mood. Some studies suggest that fasting can increase the production of brain-derived neurotrophic factor (BDNF), a protein that supports neural growth and mood regulation.

Enhanced Cognitive Function: Fasting has been shown to improve cognitive function and mental clarity, which can positively impact mood. By optimizing brain health and reducing brain fog, intermittent fasting may contribute to a more positive outlook and increased feelings of well-being.

Psychological Benefits: Intermittent fasting can have psychological benefits beyond physical health improvements. Successfully completing fasting periods and achieving weight loss goals can boost self-esteem, confidence, and feelings of accomplishment, all of which contribute to improved mood and overall well-being.

Physical Activity and Exercise

Physical activity and exercise are integral components of overall well-being, especially when combined with intermittent fasting. Physical activity, quality sleep, and adequate recovery are vital components of overall well-being, especially when combined with intermittent fasting. Seniors can safely incorporate exercise into their routine by choosing low-impact activities, listening to their bodies, and prioritizing rest and recovery. Quality sleep is essential for supporting physical and mental health, so establish a consistent sleep routine and practice relaxation techniques to improve sleep quality. By prioritizing physical activity, quality sleep, and recovery, seniors can enhance their overall well-being and maximize the benefits of intermittent fasting.

Here's how seniors can safely incorporate exercise into their routine and combine it with fasting:

Safe Exercises for Seniors

Low-Impact Activities: Opt for low-impact exercises that are gentle on the joints and suitable for seniors. Examples include walking, swimming, cycling, tai chi, yoga, and water aerobics.

Strength Training: Incorporate strength training exercises to maintain muscle mass, bone density, and functional strength. Use light weights, resistance bands, or bodyweight exercises to perform exercises targeting major muscle groups.

Flexibility and Balance: Include flexibility and balance exercises to improve mobility, posture and reduce the risk of falls. Stretching, yoga, and tai chi are excellent choices for improving flexibility and balance.

Adapted Exercises: Consider modified or adapted exercises if you have mobility limitations or health concerns. Work with a qualified fitness professional or physical therapist to create a customized exercise plan that meets your needs and abilities.

Combining Exercise with Fasting

Timing: Consider scheduling your workouts during your eating windows or shortly before breaking your fast. Exercising in a fed state can provide fuel for energy and enhance performance during workouts.

Hydration: Stay hydrated before, during, and after exercise, especially during fasting periods. Drink water or herbal tea to prevent dehydration and support optimal performance.

Listen to Your Body: Pay attention to how your body responds to exercise, particularly during fasting periods. If you feel lightheaded, dizzy, or excessively fatigued, it may be a sign that you need to adjust your exercise intensity or timing.

Post-Workout Nutrition: After completing a workout, prioritize refueling with a balanced meal containing protein, carbohydrates, and healthy fats to support muscle recovery and replenish energy stores.

Quality Sleep and Recovery

Quality sleep and adequate recovery are essential components of overall well-being, especially when practicing intermittent fasting:

Establish a Sleep Routine: Create a consistent sleep schedule by going to bed and waking up at the same time each day, even on weekends. Aim for 7-9 hours of uninterrupted sleep per night to support optimal health and well-being.

Create a Relaxing Environment: Make your bedroom conducive to sleep by keeping it dark, quiet, and cool. Limit exposure to screens (TV, phone, computer) before bedtime, as the blue light emitted can interfere with melatonin production and disrupt sleep.

Practice Relaxation Techniques: Incorporate relaxation techniques such as deep breathing, meditation, or gentle stretching before bedtime to promote relaxation and prepare your body for sleep.

Prioritize Rest and Recovery: Allow time for rest and recovery between workouts to prevent overtraining and support muscle repair. Listen to your body's signals and incorporate rest days into your exercise routine as needed.

Stay Hydrated: Drink plenty of water throughout the day to stay hydrated and support recovery processes. Dehydration can impair recovery and contribute to muscle cramps and fatigue.

Manage Stress: Practice stress management techniques such as mindfulness, meditation, or journaling to reduce stress levels and promote relaxation. Chronic stress can interfere with sleep quality and overall well-being, so it's essential to find healthy ways to cope with stress.

Seek Professional Help if Needed: If you struggle with sleep issues or chronic stress, consider seeking guidance from a healthcare professional or sleep specialist. They can provide personalized recommendations and treatments to improve sleep quality and overall well-being.

Chapter 7:

Intermittent Fasting Challenges and Solutions

Intermittent fasting can bring about various challenges, but with the right strategies, these obstacles can be overcome. Let's explore some common challenges and practical solutions:

1. **Hunger Pangs:** Feeling hungry, especially during fasting periods, is a common challenge when practicing intermittent fasting. Hunger pangs can be distracting and may tempt you to break your fast prematurely.

Solutions:
- **Stay Hydrated:** Drinking water, herbal tea, or black coffee can help curb hunger and keep you hydrated during fasting periods.

- **Fill Up on Fiber:** Include fiber-rich foods like fruits, vegetables, whole grains, and legumes in your meals to help you feel fuller for longer.

- **Chew Gum or Mints:** Sugar-free gum or mints can help reduce feelings of hunger and provide a distraction during fasting periods.

- **Practice Mindfulness:** Tune into your body's hunger signals and practice mindfulness techniques to help manage cravings and emotional eating.

- **Distraction Techniques:** Managing hunger pangs and food cravings during fasting periods can be challenging. Finding effective distraction techniques can help redirect your focus and alleviate feelings of hunger.

Engage in activities that keep your mind occupied, such as reading, hobbies, puzzles, or crafts. Keeping your hands and mind busy can help distract you from thoughts of food.

2. **Social Situations:** Navigating social situations, such as family gatherings, parties, or dinners with friends, can be challenging when practicing intermittent fasting. Peer pressure or social norms may tempt you to break your fast or indulge in unhealthy foods.

Solutions:

- **Plan Ahead:** Before attending social events, plan your fasting schedule and eating window accordingly. Adjust your fasting window or meal timing to accommodate social gatherings.

- **Communicate with Others:** Let friends and family know about your fasting routine and dietary preferences. Educate them on the benefits of intermittent fasting and ask for their support.

- **Bring Your Own Food:** If possible, bring a healthy dish or snack that aligns with your fasting goals to social gatherings. This ensures you have options available that fit your dietary preferences.

- **Focus on Socializing:** Shift the focus away from food by engaging in meaningful conversations, participating in activities, or enjoying the company of others. Remember that socializing is about more than just eating.

3. **Energy Levels:** Some individuals may experience fluctuations in energy levels, especially during the initial stages of intermittent fasting. Low energy can affect productivity, mood, and motivation to exercise.

Solutions:

- **Get Adequate Sleep:** Prioritize quality sleep to support energy levels and overall well-being. Aim for 7-9 hours of uninterrupted sleep per night to feel refreshed and energized.

- **Eat Nutrient-Dense Foods:** Focus on nutrient-dense foods that provide sustained energy throughout the day. Include complex carbohydrates, lean proteins, healthy fats, and plenty of fruits and vegetables in your meals.

- **Adjust Your Fasting Schedule:** Experiment with different fasting schedules or meal timing to find what works best for your energy levels. Some individuals may feel more energetic in the morning, while others may prefer to fast later in the day.

- **Stay Active:** Incorporate regular physical activity into your routine to boost energy levels and improve mood. Even short walks or gentle stretching can help increase circulation and alleviate feelings of fatigue.

- **Stay Hydrated:** Dehydration can contribute to feelings of fatigue, so make sure to drink plenty of water throughout the day. Herbal teas, infused water, and electrolyte-rich beverages can also help maintain hydration levels.

4. **Meal Planning:** Planning meals and snacks during eating windows can be challenging, especially if you're new to intermittent fasting or unsure of what to eat.

Practical Solutions:

- **Plan Ahead:** Take time to plan your meals and snacks for the week, considering nutrient-dense foods that align with your fasting goals. Batch cooking or meal prepping can save time and ensure you have healthy options readily available.

- **Focus on Balance:** Aim for balanced meals that include a variety of food groups, including lean proteins, complex carbohydrates, healthy fats, and plenty of fruits and vegetables. Incorporating a mix of nutrients can help keep you satisfied and energized throughout the day.

- **Choose Convenient Options:** Opt for convenient and portable meal and snack options that fit your lifestyle and schedule. Pre-packaged snacks like nuts, Greek yogurt, cut-up vegetables, or hard-boiled eggs can be convenient options for on-the-go eating.

- **Experiment with Recipes:** Get creative in the kitchen and experiment with new recipes that fit your fasting goals. Look for recipe inspiration online or in cookbooks, and don't be afraid to try new flavors and ingredients.

5.   **Staying   Motivated:** Maintaining motivation and consistency with intermittent fasting can be challenging, especially if you encounter setbacks or slow progress.

Practical Solutions:
- **Set Realistic Goals:** Establish achievable goals that are specific,

measurable, and time-bound. Break larger goals into smaller, more manageable milestones to track your progress and celebrate successes along the way.

- **Find Your Why:** Identify your reasons for practicing intermittent fasting and remind yourself of your motivations regularly. Whether you're seeking weight loss, improved health, or increased energy, connecting with your underlying why can help keep you focused and motivated.

- **Track Your Progress:** Keep track of your fasting schedule, meals, physical activity, and progress towards your goals. Use a journal, app, or calendar to monitor your achievements and identify areas for improvement.

- **Celebrate Achievements:** Acknowledge and celebrate your accomplishments, no matter how small. Reward yourself for sticking to your fasting schedule, reaching milestones, or making positive changes to your lifestyle.

- **Seek Support:** Surround yourself with a supportive community of friends, family, or online peers who understand your fasting goals and can provide encouragement, accountability, and motivation.

- **Stay Positive:** Maintain a positive mindset and focus on the progress you've made rather than dwelling on setbacks or challenges. Remember that intermittent fasting is a journey, and every step forward is a step in the right direction.

Chapter 8:

Recipes for Intermittent Fasting

1.   Healthy   Breakfasts (Post-Fasting)

Breakfast is an essential meal for breaking the fast and refueling your body after a fasting period. Here are some nutritious and delicious smoothie recipes to kickstart your day:

Green Smoothie

Ingredients:
- 1 cup spinach leaves
- 1/2 cup kale leaves
- 1/2 frozen banana
- 1/2 cup frozen mango chunks
- 1/2 cup unsweetened almond milk
- 1 tablespoon chia seeds
- 1 tablespoon honey or maple syrup (optional)
- Ice cubes (optional)

Instructions:

1. Place spinach, kale, banana, mango, almond milk, and chia seeds in a blender.

2. Blend until smooth and creamy, adding more almond milk or water if needed to reach your desired consistency.

3. Taste and adjust sweetness, if desired, by adding honey or maple syrup.

4. Pour into a glass, add ice cubes if desired, and enjoy immediately.

Berry Blast Smoothie

Ingredients:

- 1/2 cup mixed berries (such as strawberries, blueberries, raspberries)
- 1/2 frozen banana
- 1/2 cup plain Greek yogurt
- 1/2 cup unsweetened almond milk
- 1 tablespoon almond butter
- 1 tablespoon honey or maple syrup (optional)
- Ice cubes (optional)

Instructions:
1. Combine mixed berries, banana, Greek yogurt, almond milk, almond butter, and honey or maple syrup in a blender.
2. Blend until smooth and creamy, adjusting the consistency with more almond milk if needed.
3. Taste and add additional sweetener if desired.
4. Pour into a glass, add ice cubes if desired, and enjoy immediately.

<u>Tropical Smoothie</u>

Ingredients:
- 1/2 cup frozen pineapple chunks
- 1/2 frozen banana
- 1/2 cup coconut water
- 1/4 cup Greek yogurt
- 1 tablespoon shredded coconut
- 1 tablespoon lime juice
- Ice cubes (optional)

Instructions:

1. In a blender, combine frozen pineapple, banana, coconut water, Greek yogurt, shredded coconut, and lime juice.

2. Blend until smooth and creamy, adding more coconut water if needed to reach your desired consistency.

3. Taste and adjust sweetness or acidity with more lime juice or honey if desired.

4. Pour into a glass, add ice cubes if desired, and enjoy immediately.

Oatmeal Variations

Oatmeal is a versatile and nutritious breakfast option that can be customized to suit a variety of tastes and dietary preferences. Here are some delicious oatmeal variations to try:

1. Classic Oatmeal

Ingredients:
- 1/2 cup rolled oats

- 1 cup water or milk (dairy or plant-based)
- Pinch of salt
- Optional toppings: sliced banana, berries, nuts, seeds, honey or maple syrup

Instructions:
1. In a saucepan, bring water or milk to a boil.
2. Stir in rolled oats and salt, reduce heat to low, and simmer for 5-7 minutes, stirring occasionally, until oats are creamy and tender.
3. Remove from heat and let oatmeal sit for a few minutes to thicken.
4. Serve hot, topped with your favorite toppings such as sliced banana, berries, nuts, seeds, and a drizzle of honey or maple syrup.

2. Overnight Oats

Ingredients:
- 1/2 cup rolled oats

- 1/2 cup milk (dairy or plant-based)
- 1/4 cup Greek yogurt (optional, for added creaminess)
- 1 tablespoon chia seeds (optional, for added texture and nutrition)
- Optional sweetener: honey, maple syrup, or mashed banana
- Optional flavorings: vanilla extract, cinnamon, cocoa powder

Instructions:

1. In a jar or container, combine rolled oats, milk, Greek yogurt, chia seeds, sweetener, and flavorings (if using).
2. Stir well to combine, then cover and refrigerate overnight, or for at least 4 hours, to allow the oats to soften and absorb the liquid.
3. In the morning, give the oats a stir and add additional milk if desired to reach your preferred consistency.
4. Serve cold or heat in the microwave for a warm breakfast, and top with your favorite toppings such as fresh fruit, nuts, seeds, or a dollop of nut butter.

Avocado Toast

Avocado toast is a trendy and delicious breakfast option that's packed with nutrients and flavor. Here's how to make a basic avocado toast, along with some variations:

Ingredients:
- 1 ripe avocado
- 2 slices whole grain bread, toasted
- Salt and pepper to taste
- Optional toppings: sliced tomato, poached egg, microgreens, feta cheese, red pepper flakes, balsamic glaze

Instructions:
1. Cut the avocado in half, remove the pit, and scoop the flesh into a bowl.
2. Mash the avocado with a fork until smooth or slightly chunky, depending on your preference.
3. Season the mashed avocado with salt and pepper to taste.

4. Spread the mashed avocado evenly onto the toasted bread slices.
5. Top with your desired toppings, such as sliced tomato, poached egg, microgreens, feta cheese, red pepper flakes, or a drizzle of balsamic glaze.
6. Serve immediately and enjoy!

Nutritional Information and Alternatives

- Oatmeal: Oats are rich in fiber, protein, and various nutrients, including manganese, phosphorus, magnesium, and zinc. For those with gluten intolerance or celiac disease, choose certified gluten-free oats.
- Avocado Toast: Avocados are a good source of healthy fats, fiber, vitamins, and minerals, including potassium, vitamin K, vitamin E, and folate. For those with gluten intolerance, use gluten-free bread or serve the avocado mash on rice cakes or corn thins.

These oatmeal variations and avocado toast provide a nutritious and satisfying start to your day, whether you're following an intermittent fasting regimen or simply looking for a delicious breakfast option. Experiment with different toppings and flavor combinations to keep things interesting and enjoy the benefits of a wholesome morning meal!

Here are two delicious salad bowl recipes to enjoy for lunch:

1. Grilled Chicken Caesar Salad Bowl

Ingredients:
- 2 boneless, skinless chicken breasts
- 1 head romaine lettuce, chopped
- 1 cup cherry tomatoes, halved
- 1/2 cup croutons
- 1/4 cup grated Parmesan cheese
- Caesar dressing (store-bought or homemade)

Instructions:
1. Preheat the grill to medium-high heat.
2. Season the chicken breasts with salt and pepper, then grill for 6-8 minutes per side, or until cooked through.
3. Once cooked, let the chicken rest for a few minutes, then slice into strips.
4. In a large bowl, combine the chopped romaine lettuce, cherry tomatoes, croutons, and Parmesan cheese.
5. Drizzle Caesar dressing over the salad ingredients and toss to coat evenly.
6. Divide the salad mixture between two bowls and top each with sliced grilled chicken.
7. Serve immediately and enjoy your Grilled Chicken Caesar Salad Bowl!

2. Mediterranean Quinoa Salad Bowl

Ingredients:
- 1 cup cooked quinoa
- 1 cup chickpeas, drained and rinsed

- 1 cucumber, diced
- 1 cup cherry tomatoes, halved
- 1/4 cup Kalamata olives, pitted and halved
- 1/4 cup crumbled feta cheese
- 2 tablespoons chopped fresh parsley
- Juice of 1 lemon
- 2 tablespoons extra virgin olive oil
- Salt and pepper to taste

Instructions:

1. In a large bowl, combine the cooked quinoa, chickpeas, cucumber, cherry tomatoes, Kalamata olives, crumbled feta cheese, and chopped parsley.

2. In a small bowl, whisk together the lemon juice and extra virgin olive oil. Season with salt and pepper to taste.

3. Pour the dressing over the salad ingredients and toss to combine.

4. Divide the Mediterranean Quinoa Salad between two bowls.

5. Serve immediately, or refrigerate for later.

These salad bowl recipes are easy to prepare, packed with flavor, and perfect for a satisfying lunch. Feel free to customize them with your favorite ingredients and dressings to suit your taste preferences!

3. Asian-Inspired Chicken and Mango Salad Bowl

Ingredients:
- 2 boneless, skinless chicken breasts
- 1 ripe mango, peeled and diced
- 1 red bell pepper, thinly sliced
- 1/2 cup shredded carrots
- 1/4 cup chopped fresh cilantro
- 1/4 cup chopped green onions
- 1/4 cup chopped roasted peanuts or cashews
- Sesame seeds for garnish
- Optional: cooked rice noodles or quinoa for extra bulk

Dressing:
- 3 tablespoons soy sauce

- 2 tablespoons rice vinegar
- 1 tablespoon sesame oil
- 1 tablespoon honey or maple syrup
- 1 teaspoon grated ginger
- 1 garlic clove, minced

Instructions:

1. Season the chicken breasts with salt and pepper, then grill or cook them in a skillet until cooked through. Let them cool, then slice into strips.

2. In a large bowl, combine the diced mango, sliced red bell pepper, shredded carrots, chopped cilantro, and chopped green onions.

3. Add the sliced chicken to the bowl and toss everything together.

4. In a small bowl, whisk together the soy sauce, rice vinegar, sesame oil, honey or maple syrup, grated ginger, and minced garlic to make the dressing.

5. Pour the dressing over the salad ingredients and toss to coat.

6. Divide the salad between two bowls, then top each with chopped peanuts or cashews and sesame seeds.

7. Serve immediately and enjoy your Asian-Inspired Chicken and Mango Salad Bowl!

4. Greek-inspired Quinoa Salad Bowl

Ingredients:
- 1 cup cooked quinoa
- 1 cup cherry tomatoes, halved
- 1/2 cucumber, diced
- 1/4 red onion, thinly sliced
- 1/4 cup Kalamata olives, pitted and halved
- 1/4 cup crumbled feta cheese
- 2 tablespoons chopped fresh parsley
- Juice of 1 lemon
- 2 tablespoons extra virgin olive oil
- Salt and pepper to taste

Instructions:
1. In a large bowl, combine the cooked quinoa, cherry tomatoes, diced

cucumber, sliced red onion, Kalamata olives, crumbled feta cheese, and chopped parsley.

2. In a small bowl, whisk together the lemon juice and extra virgin olive oil. Season with salt and pepper to taste.

3. Pour the dressing over the salad ingredients and toss to combine.

4. Divide the Greek-inspired Quinoa Salad between two bowls.

5. Serve immediately, or refrigerate for later. Enjoy your refreshing and flavorful Greek-inspired salad bowl!

Hearty Soups

<u>1. Lentil and Vegetable Soup</u>

Ingredients:
- 1 cup dried green lentils, rinsed and drained
- 4 cups vegetable broth
- 1 onion, diced

- 2 carrots, diced
- 2 celery stalks, diced
- 2 cloves garlic, minced
- 1 can (14 oz) diced tomatoes
- 2 cups chopped kale or spinach
- 1 teaspoon dried thyme
- 1 teaspoon dried oregano
- Salt and pepper to taste
- Olive oil for cooking

Instructions:

1. Heat olive oil in a large pot over medium heat. Add diced onion, carrots, and celery, and cook until softened, about 5 minutes.

2. Add minced garlic, dried thyme, and dried oregano, and cook for another minute until fragrant.

3. Stir in diced tomatoes (with juices), rinsed lentils, and vegetable broth. Bring to a boil, then reduce heat to low and let simmer for 20-25 minutes until lentils are tender.

4. Stir in chopped kale or spinach and cook for an additional 5 minutes until wilted.

5. Season with salt and pepper to taste. Serve hot and enjoy your nutritious Lentil and Vegetable Soup!

2. Chicken and Vegetable Soup

Ingredients:
- 2 boneless, skinless chicken breasts
- 4 cups chicken broth
- 1 onion, diced
- 2 carrots, diced
- 2 celery stalks, diced
- 2 cloves garlic, minced
- 1 teaspoon dried thyme
- 1 teaspoon dried rosemary
- Salt and pepper to taste
- Olive oil for cooking

Instructions:
1. Heat olive oil in a large pot over medium heat. Add diced onion, carrots,

and celery, and cook until softened, about 5 minutes.

2. Add minced garlic, dried thyme, and dried rosemary, and cook for another minute until fragrant.

3. Add chicken breasts and chicken broth to the pot. Bring to a boil, then reduce heat to low and let simmer for 20-25 minutes until chicken is cooked through.

4. Remove chicken breasts from the pot and shred with two forks. Return shredded chicken to the pot.

5. Season with salt and pepper to taste. Serve hot and enjoy your comforting Chicken and Vegetable Soup!

Lean Protein Dishes

1. Baked Salmon with Lemon and Dill

Ingredients:
- 2 salmon fillets
- 1 lemon, sliced

- Fresh dill, chopped
- Salt and pepper to taste
- Olive oil for drizzling

Instructions:
1. Preheat the oven to 375°F (190°C). Line a baking sheet with parchment paper.
2. Place salmon fillets on the prepared baking sheet. Season with salt and pepper to taste.
3. Top each salmon fillet with lemon slices and chopped fresh dill. Drizzle with olive oil.
4. Bake in the preheated oven for 12-15 minutes, or until salmon is cooked through and flakes easily with a fork.
5. Serve hot and enjoy your flavorful Baked Salmon with Lemon and Dill!

2. Grilled Chicken with Herbs

Ingredients:
- 2 boneless, skinless chicken breasts
- 2 tablespoons olive oil

- 2 cloves garlic, minced
- 1 teaspoon dried thyme
- 1 teaspoon dried rosemary
- Salt and pepper to taste

Instructions:

1. In a small bowl, mix together olive oil, minced garlic, dried thyme, dried rosemary, salt, and pepper to make a marinade.

2. Place chicken breasts in a shallow dish or resealable plastic bag. Pour the marinade over the chicken, making sure it's evenly coated. Cover or seal and refrigerate for at least 30 minutes, or up to 4 hours.

3. Preheat grill to medium-high heat. Remove chicken from marinade and discard excess marinade.

4. Grill chicken breasts for 6-8 minutes per side, or until cooked through and no longer pink in the center.

5. Remove from grill and let rest for a few minutes before serving. Serve hot.

Dinner Recipes

1. Stir-Fried Vegetables

Ingredients:
- 2 cups mixed vegetables (such as bell peppers, broccoli, carrots, snap peas, and mushrooms), sliced or chopped
- 2 cloves garlic, minced
- 1 tablespoon sesame oil
- 2 tablespoons soy sauce (or tamari for gluten-free option)
- 1 tablespoon rice vinegar
- 1 teaspoon honey or maple syrup
- 1 tablespoon cornstarch mixed with 2 tablespoons water (optional, for thickening the sauce)
- Cooked whole grains (such as brown rice, quinoa, or farro) for serving
- Sesame seeds and sliced green onions for garnish

Instructions:
1. Heat sesame oil in a large skillet or wok over medium-high heat.

2. Add minced garlic and stir-fry for 30 seconds until fragrant.

3. Add mixed vegetables to the skillet and stir-fry for 3-5 minutes until tender-crisp.

4. In a small bowl, whisk together soy sauce, rice vinegar, and honey or maple syrup. Pour the sauce over the vegetables and toss to coat.

5. If desired, add the cornstarch-water mixture to the skillet and stir until the sauce thickens slightly.

6. Serve the stir-fried vegetables over cooked whole grains, such as brown rice, quinoa, or farro.

7. Garnish with sesame seeds and sliced green onions.

Nutritional Information: This recipe provides a good balance of carbohydrates, protein, and fiber. It's rich in vitamins, minerals, and antioxidants from the colorful array of vegetables. To reduce sodium intake, opt for low-sodium soy sauce or tamari.

Dietary Restriction Alternatives:
Gluten-Free: Use tamari instead of soy sauce to make the dish gluten-free.
Vegetarian/Vegan: Omit honey or use a plant-based sweetener to make the dish vegan. Add tofu or tempeh for extra protein.
Low-Carb: Serve the stir-fried vegetables over cauliflower rice or zucchini noodles instead of whole grains.

2. Baked Fish/Chicken

Ingredients:
- 2 fish fillets (such as salmon, cod, or tilapia) or 2 boneless, skinless chicken breasts
- 2 tablespoons olive oil
- 1 lemon, sliced
- 2 cloves garlic, minced
- Salt and pepper to taste
- Fresh herbs (such as thyme, rosemary, or dill) for garnish

Instructions:

1. Preheat the oven to 375°F (190°C). Line a baking sheet with parchment paper.

2. Place fish fillets or chicken breasts on the prepared baking sheet.

3. Drizzle olive oil over the fish/chicken and season with minced garlic, salt, and pepper.

4. Top each fillet or breast with lemon slices and fresh herbs.

5. Bake in the preheated oven for 12-15 minutes for fish, or 20-25 minutes for chicken, or until cooked through and tender.

6. Serve hot with your choice of cooked whole grains and steamed vegetables. Enjoy your flavorful Baked Fish/Chicken!

Nutritional Information: This recipe is rich in protein and healthy fats (for fish), providing essential nutrients like omega-3 fatty acids (found in fatty fish like salmon). For chicken, it's a lean protein source. The dish is low in carbohydrates and can be paired with whole grains for a balanced meal.

Dietary Restriction Alternatives:
Low-Carb: Serve the baked fish/chicken with a side of roasted vegetables or a salad instead of whole grains for a lower-carb option.

3. Whole Grain Pilaf

Ingredients:
- 1 cup whole grains (such as brown rice, quinoa, farro, or barley)
- 2 cups vegetable or chicken broth
- 1 tablespoon olive oil
- 1 onion, diced
- 2 cloves garlic, minced
- 1 carrot, diced
- 1 celery stalk, diced
- 1/4 cup chopped parsley
- Salt and pepper to taste

Instructions:

1. In a saucepan, heat olive oil over medium heat. Add diced onion, minced garlic, diced carrot, and diced celery, and sauté until softened, about 5 minutes.

2. Add whole grains to the saucepan and toast for 2-3 minutes, stirring frequently.

3. Pour vegetable or chicken broth into the saucepan and bring to a boil.

4. Reduce heat to low, cover, and simmer for 20-25 minutes, or until the grains are tender and liquid is absorbed.

5. Remove from heat and let the pilaf sit, covered, for 5 minutes. Fluff with a fork

Snack Options

1. Mixed Nuts and Seeds

Ingredients:

- 1/4 cup mixed nuts (such as almonds, walnuts, cashews, and pistachios)

- 2 tablespoons mixed seeds (such as pumpkin seeds, sunflower seeds, and chia seeds)
- Optional: a pinch of salt or your favorite spices (such as cinnamon or paprika)

Instructions:
1. Combine mixed nuts and seeds in a small bowl.
2. If desired, sprinkle with a pinch of salt or your favorite spices for extra flavor.
3. Toss to combine.
4. Portion into individual snack bags or containers for easy grab-and-go snacking.
5. Enjoy your crunchy and nutritious Mixed Nuts and Seeds snack!

Nutritional Information: This snack is rich in healthy fats, protein, fiber, vitamins, and minerals from the nuts and seeds. It provides sustained energy and helps keep you feeling full and satisfied between meals.

Dietary Restriction Alternatives:
Nut-Free: Substitute nuts with roasted chickpeas or roasted edamame for a crunchy snack option.
Seed-Free: Omit seeds or replace them with additional nuts or dried fruits if you have seed allergies or sensitivities.

2. Fresh Fruit Salad

Ingredients:
- Assorted fresh fruits (such as strawberries, blueberries, raspberries, blackberries, grapes, kiwi, pineapple, mango, and melon), washed and chopped.
- Optional: a squeeze of lemon juice or a drizzle of honey (optional for added flavor)

Instructions:
1. Wash and chop assorted fresh fruits of your choice and place them in a large bowl.

2. If desired, add a squeeze of lemon juice or a drizzle of honey for extra flavor.

3. Gently toss to combine.

4. Portion into individual serving bowls or containers for easy snacking.

5. Enjoy your refreshing and vitamin-packed Fresh Fruit Salad!

Nutritional Information: This snack is packed with vitamins, minerals, fiber, and antioxidants from a variety of fresh fruits. It's low in calories and provides natural sweetness and hydration.

Dietary Restriction Alternatives:

Low-Sugar: Choose lower-sugar fruits such as berries, kiwi, and melon to reduce overall sugar content.

Citrus-Free: Omit citrus fruits if you have citrus allergies or sensitivities.

<u>3. Yogurt with Berries</u>

Ingredients:

- 1/2 cup plain Greek yogurt (or dairy-free yogurt for a vegan option)
- 1/2 cup mixed berries (such as strawberries, blueberries, raspberries, and blackberries)
- Optional: a drizzle of honey or maple syrup for sweetness

Instructions:

1. Spoon plain Greek yogurt into a serving bowl.
2. Top with mixed berries.
3. If desired, drizzle with honey or maple syrup for added sweetness.
4. Enjoy your creamy and antioxidant-rich Yogurt with Berries!

Nutritional Information: This snack is high in protein, probiotics (if using yogurt with live cultures), vitamins, minerals, and antioxidants from Greek yogurt and mixed berries. It provides a satisfying and nourishing snack option.

Dietary Restriction Alternatives:
Vegan: Use dairy-free yogurt made from soy, almond, coconut, or oat milk for a vegan option.
Low-Fat: Choose low-fat or fat-free yogurt for a lower-fat option.

Chapter 9

Testimonials

Emily's Weight Loss Journey:
"After struggling with weight gain for years, I decided to try intermittent fasting. With the 16/8 method, I restricted my eating window to 8 hours a day. Within a few months, I lost 20 pounds and regained my confidence. Intermittent fasting not only helped me shed excess weight but also improved my energy levels and overall well-being."

Mark's Metabolic Transformation:
"As a diabetic, I was skeptical about intermittent fasting at first. But after consulting with my doctor, I decided to give it a try. With careful monitoring and adjustments to my medication, I adopted the 5:2 diet, fasting for two non-consecutive days a week. Over time, my blood sugar levels stabilized, and I

was able to reduce my reliance on insulin. Intermittent fasting has been a game-changer for managing my diabetes."

Sarah's Social Dilemma:
"One of the biggest challenges I faced with intermittent fasting was social gatherings and events. It was tough to stick to my fasting schedule while everyone around me was enjoying food and drinks. But with support from friends and family, I found ways to navigate social situations without compromising my fasting goals. Planning ahead, staying hydrated, and focusing on socializing rather than food helped me overcome this hurdle."

John's Hunger Management:
"During the initial stages of intermittent fasting, I struggled with intense hunger pangs, especially in the mornings. It took time for my body to adjust to the new eating pattern. To overcome this

challenge, I experimented with different fasting methods and gradually extended my fasting window. Incorporating more fiber-rich foods and staying hydrated helped curb hunger and keep me on track with my fasting goals."

3. Expert Opinions

Dr. Maya Patel, Nutritionist:
"Intermittent fasting has gained popularity for its potential health benefits, including weight loss, improved metabolic health, and longevity. Research suggests that intermittent fasting may promote cellular repair processes, enhance insulin sensitivity, and reduce inflammation. However, it's important to approach intermittent fasting with caution and consult with a healthcare professional, especially for individuals with underlying medical conditions."

Professor David Wong, Endocrinologist:

"While intermittent fasting shows promise for improving metabolic health and weight management, it's not a one-size-fits-all approach. Different fasting methods may work better for different individuals, and adherence is key for long-term success. It's essential to prioritize nutrient-dense foods during eating windows and avoid compensatory overeating. Overall, intermittent fasting can be a valuable tool when incorporated into a balanced lifestyle."

These personal stories and expert opinions provide valuable insights into the experiences, challenges, and benefits of intermittent fasting. From weight loss success to overcoming hurdles and expert advice, individuals can find inspiration and guidance on their own intermittent fasting journey.

CONCLUSION

Summary of Key Points

In this book, we've explored the principles and practices of intermittent fasting, uncovering its potential benefits for weight loss, metabolic health, and overall well-being. From understanding different fasting methods to exploring the science behind fasting, readers have gained valuable insights into this lifestyle approach to nutrition.

Encouragement to Start

Embarking on the journey of intermittent fasting can be both exciting and challenging, but the rewards are worth it. Whether you're looking to shed excess weight, improve metabolic health, or simply adopt a healthier lifestyle, intermittent fasting offers a flexible and sustainable approach. Remember that every journey begins with a single step, and with determination, patience, and support, you can achieve your health goals through intermittent fasting.

APPENDICES

Glossary of Terms

Intermittent Fasting: A dietary pattern that involves alternating periods of fasting and eating.

Eating Window: The designated time period during which one consumes food within an intermittent fasting regimen.

Fasting Window: The designated time period during which one abstains from consuming food within an intermittent fasting regimen.

16/8 Method: A form of intermittent fasting where one fasts for 16 hours and consumes all meals within an 8-hour window.

5:2 Diet: An intermittent fasting approach where one eats normally for five days of the week and restricts calorie intake on the remaining two days.

Eat-Stop-Eat: An intermittent fasting method that involves fasting for 24 hours once or twice a week.

Alternate-Day Fasting: A fasting approach where one alternates between fasting days and non-fasting days.

Metabolic Health: The state of optimal metabolic function, including factors such as blood sugar regulation, cholesterol levels, and blood pressure.

Insulin Sensitivity: The body's ability to respond to insulin and regulate blood sugar levels effectively.

Cellular Repair Processes: Mechanisms within the body that repair damaged cells and promote overall cellular health.

Inflammation: The body's immune response to injury, infection, or stress, which can contribute to various health conditions if chronic.

Lean Proteins: Protein sources that are low in fat content, such as chicken breast, turkey, fish, tofu, and legumes.

Whole Grains: Grains that retain all parts of the grain kernel, including the bran, germ, and endosperm, such as brown rice, quinoa, barley, and oats.

Frequently Asked Questions

1. Is intermittent fasting safe for seniors?

- Intermittent fasting can be safe for seniors when done properly and under the guidance of a healthcare professional. It's essential to consider individual health conditions and nutritional needs.

2. What can I consume during fasting hours?

- During fasting hours, it's typically recommended to consume only non-caloric beverages such as water, herbal tea, black coffee, or sparkling water.

3. Will intermittent fasting help me lose weight?

- Intermittent fasting can be an effective tool for weight loss by promoting a calorie deficit and enhancing fat burning. However, individual results may vary, and consistency is key.

4. How should I break my fast?

- It's important to break your fast with nutrient-dense, balanced meals containing protein, healthy fats, and carbohydrates. Avoiding excessive processed foods and sugars is advisable.

5. Can I exercise while fasting?

- Moderate exercise during fasting hours is generally safe and may even enhance the benefits of intermittent fasting. However, listen to your body and adjust your activity level accordingly.

This 1-month exercise challenge is designed to help seniors improve their overall fitness, strength, and mobility. The program includes a mix of cardiovascular exercises, strength training, balance exercises, and flexibility routines. Always consult your doctor before starting any new exercise program, especially if you have any preexisting health conditions.

Week 1: Building the Foundation

1 Month Exercise Challenge for Seniors

Week 1:
Building the Foundation

DAY 1

Walking and Stretching
Activity: 20-minute brisk
walk
- Stretching: 5-10 minutes of
gentle stretching (focus on
legs, arms, and back)

DAY 2

Strength Training
- Exercises:
- Chair Squats: 2 sets of 10 reps
- Wall Push-Ups: 2 sets of 10 reps
- Bicep Curls with Light Weights or
Resistance Bands: 2 sets of 10 reps

DAY 3

Balance and Flexibility
- Exercises:
- Standing on One Leg: 2 sets of 15
seconds each leg
- Heel-to-Toe Walk: 2 sets of 20 steps
- Stretching: 5-10 minutes

DAY 4

Rest and Recovery
- Activity: Gentle stretching or
yoga

DAY 5

Cardio and Strength
- Activity: 15-minute walk
- Strength Exercises:
- Seated Leg Lifts: 2 sets of 10 reps each
leg
- Overhead Press with Light Weights: 2
sets of 10 reps

DAY 6

Flexibility and Balance
- Exercises:
- Calf Raises: 2 sets of 10 reps
- Side Leg Raises: 2 sets of 10
reps each leg
- Stretching: 5-10 minutes

DAY 7

Rest and Gentle Activity
- Activity: Light
stretching or a leisurely
walk

1 MONTH EXERCISE CHALLENGE FOR SENIORS

Week 2:
Increasing Intensity

DAY 8

Walking and Strength
- Activity: 25-minute brisk walk
- Strength Exercises:
- Chair Squats: 2 sets of 12 reps
- Wall Push-Ups: 2 sets of 12 reps

DAY 9

Cardio and Flexibility
- Activity: 20-minute low-impact cardio (e.g., marching in place, stepping side to side)
- Stretching: 5-10 minutes

DAY 10

Strength and Balance
- Exercises:
- Bicep Curls: 2 sets of 12 reps
- Side Leg Raises: 2 sets of 12 reps each leg
- Standing on One Leg: 2 sets of 20 seconds each leg

DAY 11

Rest and Recovery
- Activity: Gentle stretching or yoga

DAY 12

Walking and Strength
- Activity: 30-minute brisk walk
- Strength Exercises:
- Seated Leg Lifts: 2 sets of 12 reps each leg
- Overhead Press: 2 sets of 12 reps

DAY 13

Balance and Flexibility
- Exercises:
- Heel-to-Toe Walk: 2 sets of 25 steps
- Calf Raises: 2 sets of 12 reps
- Stretching: 5-10 minutes

DAY 14

Rest and Gentle Activity
- Activity: Light stretching or a leisurely walk

<u>Week 3: Building Strength and Endurance</u>

1 MONTH EXERCISE CHALLENGE FOR SENIORS

<u>Week 3:</u>
<u>Building Strength and Endurance</u>

DAY 15

Walking and Strength
- Activity: 35-minute brisk walk
- Strength Exercises:
- Chair Squats: 2 sets of 15 reps
- Wall Push-Ups: 2 sets of 15 reps

DAY 16

Cardio and Flexibility
- Activity: 25-minute low-impact cardio (e.g., dancing, water aerobics)
- Stretching: 5-10 minutes

DAY 17

Strength and Balance
- Exercises:
- Bicep Curls: 2 sets of 15 reps
- Side Leg Raises: 2 sets of 15 reps each leg
- Standing on One Leg: 2 sets of 25 seconds each leg

DAY 18

Rest and Recovery
- Activity: Gentle stretching or yoga

DAY 19

Walking and Strength
- Activity: 40-minute brisk walk
- Strength Exercises:
- Seated Leg Lifts: 2 sets of 15 reps each leg
- Overhead Press: 2 sets of 15 reps

DAY 20

Balance and Flexibility
- Exercises:
- Heel-to-Toe Walk: 2 sets of 30 steps
- Calf Raises: 2 sets of 15 reps
- Stretching: 5-10 minutes

DAY 21

Rest and Gentle Activity
- Activity: Light stretching or a leisurely walk

Week 4: Maximizing Benefits

1 MONTH EXERCISE CHALLENGE FOR SENIORS

Week 4:
Maximizing Benefits

DAY 22

Walking and Strength
- Activity: 45-minute brisk walk
- Strength Exercises:
- Chair Squats: 2 sets of 15 reps
- Wall Push-Ups: 2 sets of 15 reps

DAY 23

Cardio and Flexibility
- Activity: 25-minute low-impact cardio (e.g., dancing, water aerobics)
- Stretching: 5-10 minutes

DAY 24

Strength and Balance
- Exercises:
- Bicep Curls: 2 sets of 15 reps
- Side Leg Raises: 2 sets of 15 reps each leg
- Standing on One Leg: 2 sets of 30 seconds each leg

DAY 25

Rest and Recovery
- Activity: Gentle stretching or yoga

DAY 26

Walking and Strength
- Activity: 50-minute brisk walk
- Strength Exercises:
- Seated Leg Lifts: 2 sets of 15 reps each leg
- Overhead Press: 2 sets of 15 reps

DAY 27

Balance and Flexibility
- Exercises:
- Heel-to-Toe Walk: 2 sets of 30 steps
- Calf Raises: 2 sets of 15 reps
- Stretching: 5-10 minutes

DAY 28

Rest and Gentle Activity
- Activity: Light stretching or a leisurely walk

Day 29: Walking and Strength	Day 30: Cardio and Flexibility
- Activity: 55-minute brisk walk - Strength Exercises: - Chair Squats: 2 sets of 15 reps - Wall Push-Ups: 2 sets of 15 reps	- Activity: 30-minute low-impact cardio (e.g., dancing, water aerobics) - Stretching: 5-10 minutes

Final Tips

- **Stay Consistent:** Try to stick to the schedule as much as possible, but listen to your body and rest if you need to.
- **Hydrate**: Drink plenty of water throughout the day, especially before and after exercises.
- **Warm-Up and Cool Down**: Always start with a light warm-up

and end with a cool-down stretch to prevent injuries.

- **Modify as Needed:** Adjust exercises to your fitness level. If any movement causes pain, stop and consult a professional.

This challenge aims to progressively build your strength, endurance, and flexibility, setting a solid foundation for ongoing physical activity and health. Enjoy the process and celebrate your progress!

www.ingramcontent.com/pod-product-compliance
Lightning Source LLC
Chambersburg PA
CBHW012257240726
48656CB00007B/2417